Dementia Sucks

But Life Doesn't Have To

A Guided Journal for
Caregivers of Dementia
and Alzheimer's Patients

Dementia Sucks

But Life Doesn't Have To

A Guided Journal for
Caregivers of Dementia
and Alzheimer's Patients

Deborah L Mills

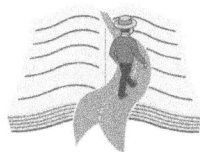

WALKER LAYNE
GROUP

Dementia Sucks
But Life Doesn't Have To
A Guided Journal for Caregivers
of Dementia and Alzheimer's Patients

ISBN 978-1-7361800-2-0 (sc)
ISBN 978-1-7361800-5-1 (hc)

Walker Layne Group, LLC walkerlaynegroup.com

This work is based on the author's experience and is not intended to act as or substitute for medical advice.

For bulk purchases, author interviews, speaking engagements and more contact the publisher.

As I walk this journey with you, I challenge you to continue to live and enjoy life. I challenge myself to do the same.

– **Deborah** ❤

Write down several memorable moments you had with your loved one that you never want to forget. Be as detailed as possible.

LIFE
IS
GOOD

What did your loved one do this week that could have caused embarressment? How did you respond? Try not to be embarressed by your loved one's actions. Choose these times to build your resilence and humor. It can also be an opportunity to educate those around you.

LIFE
IS
GOOD

How can you help to ensure you are physically protected? Loved ones with dementia may not realize their strength and are sometimes uncontrolled in their behaviors. For example, you may need to remove all knives from the kitchen or all hunting guns from the house.

LIFE
IS
GOOD

Are you experiencing grief? You may begin to experience grief now. Witnessing a negative decline can do this to you. Write down your thoughts and feelings so you can better deal with and explore them.

LIFE
IS
GOOD

What can you do that inspires happiness in your day? Write it down and then carry it out. Happiness is because of happenings, so create some happy moments.

LIFE
IS
GOOD

When is the last time you had a good belly laugh? Write down exactly what happened and why it was so funny. Laughter can be good medicine.

LIFE
IS
GOOD

Write down how you are experiencing joy even amid this challenge. Joy is an internal position that allows you to operate in peace with a smile, even when the world feels hard.

LIFE
IS
GOOD

How do you lift yourself up once the tears come or anger is present? Write it down or, if needed, take the time to figure it out.
Visit this page often.

LIFE
IS
GOOD

Write down the good, lovely, and pleasant parts of your day. Every day you will have to deal with the reality of of what is going on with this disease. However, you can focus on what is good, lovely, and pleasant.

LIFE
IS
GOOD

Feeling left out? As everyone continues with their lives, you may feel yours is standing still as a caregiver. Decide how you will involve yourself in life, family events, work events, entrepreneurship, etc. Choose what you want to be involved in and go for it. Write it down.

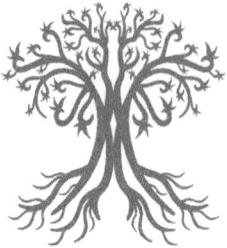

LIFE
IS
GOOD

What can you implement to focus on the celebration of life versus the task of doing? Let everyday be a celebration of life.

_____

_____

_____

_____

_____

_____

_____

_____

_____

_____

_____

_____

_____

_____

_____

LIFE
IS
GOOD

Discover something new about your loved one. If they are unable to answer questions, call a family member or do some research. Write down what you learn.

LIFE
IS
GOOD

What do you think would make your life easier right now? Write it down and implement what you can. Ask for help where needed.

LIFE
IS
GOOD

What special moments can you share with your loved one now? It's never too late to create new memories.

LIFE
IS
GOOD

Write down areas where you can display greater patience. Be patient with yourself and your loved one. You are both going through new experiences.

LIFE
IS
GOOD

What brings you calm and peace? Make a list of 10 to 15 things. Now decide what to enact first.

LIFE
IS
GOOD

What routines are you holding on to that you should release because they no longer make sense given your current situation? Are you willing to create a new routine?

LIFE
IS
GOOD

What decision have you been procrastinating on making? What's holding you up? Be honest. What's your next step and when will you complete it?

LIFE
IS
GOOD

What can you celebrate today? Write it down and keep your focus there.

LIFE
IS
GOOD

Reminisce on the good times. Take yourself down memory lane. Write it down. Capture the memory.

LIFE
IS
GOOD

How are you feeling today? Your loved one's diagnosis of dementia can stir up many emotions.

_____

_____

_____

_____

_____

_____

_____

_____

_____

_____

_____

_____

_____

LIFE
IS
GOOD

Think about and write down who will be on your team and why. The journey of dementia with your loved one will require a team.

_____
_____
_____
_____
_____
_____
_____
_____
_____
_____
_____
_____
_____
_____
_____

LIFE
IS
GOOD

Where do you need to say no? Write it down. Then write the word NO over and over and say it aloud. Caregivers tend to be loving people who want to help everyone. Sometimes you need to say no.

LIFE
IS
GOOD

What will your simple pleasure be for today, tomorrow, next week? Remember the simple pleasures you used to enjoy. Write them down and begin to enjoy them again.

Do you have boundaries for your loved one, your family, your friends, or for yourself? Write them down. Remember what you said. Boundaries are necessary for your well-being.

_____

_____

_____

_____

_____

_____

_____

_____

_____

_____

_____

_____

_____

LIFE
IS
GOOD

What have you learned through the process of caring for your loved one?

LIFE
IS
GOOD

How are you stronger today than you were yesterday?

LIFE
IS
GOOD

What do you know about yourself that you didn't know before you became a caregiver?

LIFE
IS
GOOD

How are you feeling today? Although life is not run by feelings, feelings are very real. They need to be acknowledged and understood.

Make a list of fun and adventurous things to do. Choose one and do it. The logistics may be greater now that you are a caregiver, but it's not impossible.

LIFE
IS
GOOD

How can you take better care of yourself? As a caregiver you may place yourself last. Let's move you up higher on the list. When you are well cared for, it is easier for you to take care of your loved one.

LIFE
IS
GOOD

Write down your morning routine. If you don't have one, use this space to create one and be sure to follow it. It will help you feel in control as well as start your day with less stress. Remember to be flexible. Your loved one's needs can be unpredictable.

LIFE
IS
GOOD

What is your nighttime routine? Write it down. If you don't have one, use this space to create one. Be patient with yourself and your loved one as you implement your routine. You will be a better caregiver if you are well rested.

LIFE
IS
GOOD

What made you smile today? Capture the
moment. Visit this memory often.

LIFE
IS
GOOD

Write down specific areas where you need to release the pressure of being a caregiver. Then let it go. You can only do your best.

LIFE
IS
GOOD

Write down your position of faith and belief on this journey. If you need to, seek counsel.

How can you make tomorrow better than today?

LIFE
IS
GOOD

How are you honored to care for your loved one? The mindset of "I have to take care of this person" versus "I'm honored I get to care for this person" is very different.

LIFE
IS
GOOD

Where is your mental happy place? Is it a
song? A memory? A Scripture or prayer?
Write it down. Visit it often.

_____

_____

_____

_____

_____

_____

_____

_____

_____

_____

_____

_____

_____

LIFE
IS
GOOD

What healthy stress relievers are a part of your daily routine? If you don't have any, take a moment to research some and jot them down.

LIFE
IS
GOOD

Where do you need to acknowledge your accomplishments? Write it down. When you are doing your best, remove guilt, shame, and feelings that you could do more. Give yourself credit for doing your best, even in the tough moments.

LIFE
IS
GOOD

What changes can you implement to make this experience the best it can be for you and your loved one?

LIFE
IS
GOOD

How is your family a help in this matter?
Write these ways down, however big or
small, and be grateful.

_____

_____

_____

_____

_____

_____

_____

_____

_____

_____

_____

_____

_____

_____

_____

LIFE
IS
GOOD

How is caregiving rewarding? Being a caregiver is both rewarding and tough, but let's focus on the positive today.

LIFE
IS
GOOD

Where do you see grace showing up in
this journey?

_____

_____

_____

_____

_____

_____

_____

_____

_____

_____

_____

_____

_____

LIFE
IS
GOOD

If you were not caring for your loved one what would you do with your time? Write these activities down. Plan to incorporate a few of these things in your life.

LIFE
IS
GOOD

How can you remain present in your own life during this time? As a caregiver, it's easy to get lost in the needs of your loved one.

LIFE
IS
GOOD

Make two lists. A list of words that positively describe you. The other list will positively describe your loved one. Write at least 20 words on each list. Take all the time you need but don't quit. Refer to your list often.

LIFE
IS
GOOD

What questions do you need to ask today and of whom? Write down the questions and the names of family, friends, doctors, or agencies that you need to ask.

LIFE
IS
GOOD

What do you need right now? How can you incorporate your needs into your regular schedule?

_____

_____

_____

_____

_____

_____

_____

_____

_____

_____

_____

_____

_____

_____

LIFE
IS
GOOD

How have you shown yourself love today? Your life is important and valuable. If you don't have an answer, plan now and write it down tomorrow.

LIFE
IS
GOOD

All forms of dementia suck. Let's continue to believe and pray for a cure. One day our world will be free of such horrors.

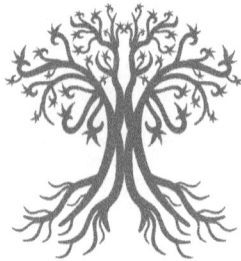

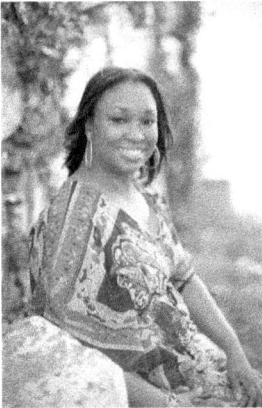

Deborah L Mills is a wife, mother, and grandmother. She enjoys writing and reading. She also likes to play with her grandchildren as often as possible. Deborah is caregiver for her mother who received a diagnosis of dementia and then Alzheimer's Disease, almost two decades ago. Alzheimer's and dementia are rising challenges that affect many families across the world.

Deborah is a certified life coach and mentor. She has a heart to see people succeed. Deborah is thrilled to share her life experiences with you in hopes that this journal will bring a ray of sunshine and hope along your journey.